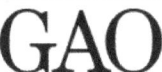

January 2012

ANTIBIOTICS

FDA Needs to Do More to Ensure That Drug Labels Contain Up-to-Date Information

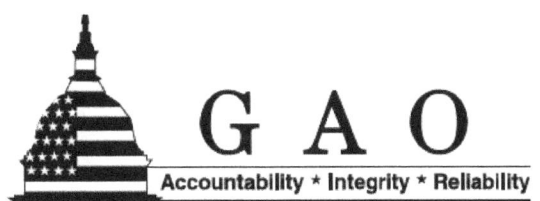
GAO
Accountability ★ Integrity ★ Reliability

GAO-12-218

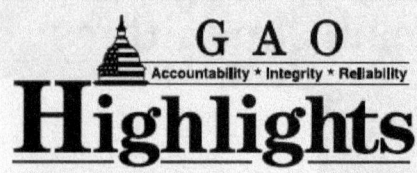
January 2012

ANTIBIOTICS

FDA Needs to Do More to Ensure That Drug Labels Contain Up-to-Date Information

Why GAO Did This Study

Antibiotics are critical drugs that have saved millions of lives. Growing bacterial resistance to existing drugs and the fact that few new drugs are in development are public health concerns. The Food and Drug Administration Amendments Act of 2007 (FDAAA) required the Food and Drug Administration (FDA), an agency within the Department of Health and Human Services (HHS), to identify, periodically update, and make publicly available up-to-date breakpoints, the concentrations at which bacteria are categorized as susceptible to an antibiotic. Breakpoints are a required part of an antibiotic's label and are used by providers to determine appropriate treatments. FDAAA provided a financial incentive for antibiotic innovation and required FDA to hold a public meeting on antibiotic incentives and innovation. FDAAA directed GAO to report on the impact of these provisions on new drugs. This report (1) assesses FDA's efforts to help preserve antibiotic effectiveness by ensuring breakpoints on labels are up to date and (2) examines the impact of the antibiotic innovation provisions. GAO examined FDA data, guidance, and other documents; interviewed FDA officials; and obtained information from drug sponsors, such as manufacturers, that market antibiotics.

What GAO Recommends

GAO recommends that the Commissioner of FDA take steps to help ensure antibiotic labels contain up-to-date information, such as by expediting the agency's review of breakpoint submissions. HHS said it will consider implementing GAO's recommendations.

View GAO-12-218. For more information, contact Marcia Crosse at (202) 512-7114 or crossem@gao.gov.

What GAO Found

FDA has not taken sufficient steps to ensure that antibiotic labels contain up-to-date breakpoints. FDA designates certain drugs as "reference-listed drugs" and the sponsors of these drugs play an important role in ensuring the accuracy of drug labels. Reference-listed drugs are approved drug products to which generic versions are compared. As of November 2011, FDA had not yet confirmed whether the breakpoints on the majority of reference-listed antibiotics labels were up to date. FDA contacted sponsors of 210 antibiotics in early 2008 to remind sponsors of the importance of maintaining their labels and requested that they assess whether the breakpoints on their drugs' labels were up to date. Sponsors were asked to submit evidence to FDA showing that the breakpoints were either current or needed revision. As of November 2011, over 3.5 years after FDA contacted sponsors, the agency had not yet confirmed whether the breakpoints on the labels of 70 percent, or 146 of the 210 antibiotics, were up to date. FDA has not ensured that sponsors have fulfilled the responsibilities outlined in the early 2008 letters. For those submissions FDA has received, it has often taken over a year for FDA to complete its review. Officials attributed this delay to reviewers' workload, challenging scientific issues or difficulties in obtaining needed data, and incomplete submissions. FDA also issued guidance to clarify sponsors' responsibility to evaluate and maintain up-to-date breakpoints. The guidance reminded sponsors that they are required to maintain accurate labels and stated that certain sponsors should submit an evaluation of breakpoints on their antibiotic labels to FDA annually. However, FDA has not been systematically tracking whether sponsors are providing these annual updates. Some sponsors remain confused about their responsibility to evaluate and maintain up-to-date breakpoints. At GAO's request, FDA reviewed a small sample of annual reports and determined that few sponsors appear to be responsive to the guidance.

The FDAAA provisions related to antibiotic innovation have not resulted in the submission of new drug applications for antibiotics. FDAAA extended the period of time that sponsors of new drugs that meet certain criteria have exclusive right to market the drug. According to FDA officials, the agency has received very few inquiries regarding this provision and, as of November 2011, no new drug applications for antibiotics have been submitted that would qualify for this exclusivity. None of the drug sponsors GAO received comments from said that this provision provided sufficient incentive to develop a new antibiotic of this type. FDAAA also required that FDA hold a public meeting to discuss whether and how existing or potential incentives could be applied to promote the development of antibiotics. Both financial and regulatory incentives were discussed at FDA's 2008 meeting, including tax incentives for research and development and providing greater regulatory clarity during the drug approval process.

_____ United States Government Accountability Office

Contents

Abbreviations

ANDA	abbreviated new drug application
FDA	Food and Drug Administration
FDAAA	Food and Drug Administration Amendments Act of 2007
HHS	Department of Health and Human Services
NDA	new drug application
NME	new molecular entity

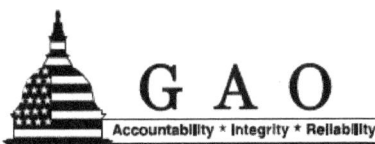

United States Government Accountability Office
Washington, DC 20548

January 31, 2012

The Honorable Tom Harkin
Chairman
The Honorable Michael B. Enzi
Ranking Member
Committee on Health, Education, Labor, and Pensions
United States Senate

The Honorable Fred Upton
Chairman
The Honorable Henry A. Waxman
Ranking Member
Committee on Energy and Commerce
House of Representatives

Since the discovery of penicillin in 1928, antibiotics have played an important role in the care and well-being of people around the world. By destroying bacteria or inhibiting their growth in individuals with serious or potentially serious infections, antibiotics have saved millions of lives. Today, however, bacteria that cause serious infections in the United States and elsewhere are becoming resistant to antibiotics, making infections that once responded to these drugs more difficult to treat.[1] Meanwhile, the number of new antibiotics has steadily decreased since the 1980s.[2] The limited number of antibiotics under development is a matter of concern for the Food and Drug Administration (FDA), the agency within the Department of Health and Human Services (HHS) responsible for overseeing the safety and effectiveness of drugs marketed in the United States. The Commissioner of FDA recently

---

[1]Scientists, public health officials, and clinicians agree that antibiotic resistance has become a national and global health challenge. This resistance is a natural phenomenon caused by a variety of factors, including the inappropriate or prolonged use of antibiotics. We recently reported on antibiotic resistance. See GAO, *Antibiotic Resistance: Data Gaps Will Remain Despite HHS Taking Steps to Improve Monitoring*, GAO-11-406 (Washington, D.C.: June 1, 2011), and *Antibiotic Resistance: Agencies Have Made Limited Progress Addressing Antibiotic Use in Animals*, GAO-11-801 (Washington, D.C.: Sept. 7, 2011).

[2]H.W. Boucher, et.al., *Bad Bugs, No Drugs: No ESKAPE! An Update from the Infectious Diseases Society of America* (Arlington, Va.: Clinical Infectious Diseases, 2009).

reported that the drug pipeline is "distressingly devoid" of new antibiotics,[3] and the scientific community recognizes the lack of new antibiotics in development as a significant concern.

The development of new drugs, including antibiotics, is often a costly and lengthy process; to obtain FDA's approval to market a new drug, a sponsor must conduct extensive research in order to demonstrate that a new drug is both safe and effective.[4] Although high costs and failure rates make drug development risky for drug sponsors, creating a safe and effective new drug can be financially rewarding for the drug sponsor and beneficial to the public. However, antibiotics are often less profitable than other drugs because they are designed to work quickly and are typically administered for a brief duration. This makes them less lucrative investments for sponsors than drugs that treat chronic conditions, such as diabetes and arthritis, which may be taken for an extended period of time or even indefinitely. In addition, given the growing problem of resistance, an antibiotic may not remain effective long enough to produce a meaningful return on a sponsor's investment.[5]

Maintaining the effectiveness of antibiotics, and the need for innovation, was addressed in several provisions of the Food and Drug Administration Amendments Act of 2007 (FDAAA). Regarding the effectiveness of antibiotics already on the market, FDAAA required FDA to identify, periodically update, and make publicly available, such as on the Internet, up-to-date antibiotic "breakpoints," which are included on an antibiotic's label and reflect the concentrations at which bacteria are categorized as susceptible to treatment with a given antibiotic. Labels that contain up-to-date breakpoints are considered to be as accurate as possible and are used by health care providers to help determine the best antibiotic to treat a particular bacterial infection. Out-of-date breakpoints on antibiotic labels can result in providers unknowingly selecting ineffective antibiotic

---

[3]M.A. Hamburg, M.D., "FDA's Efforts to Facilitate Antibiotic Approvals," *Infectious Diseases Society of America World Health Day Event*, (Washington, D.C.: Apr. 7, 2011).

[4]A drug sponsor is the person or entity that assumes responsibility for the marketing of a new drug, including responsibility for complying with applicable provisions of laws, such as the Federal Food, Drug, and Cosmetic Act and related regulations. The sponsor is usually an individual, partnership, corporation, government agency, manufacturer, or scientific institution.

[5]*Bad Bugs, No Drugs: As Antibiotic Discovery Stagnates…A Public Health Crisis Brews* (Alexandria, Va.: Infectious Diseases Society of America, 2004).

treatments, which can contribute to additional bacterial resistance to antibiotics. An antibiotic's breakpoint, along with other information, is a required part of a drug's label. However, determining whether a breakpoint has changed can be complex and scientifically challenging. FDA has found it difficult to ensure that sponsors maintain labels on antibiotics that contain up-to-date breakpoints. Regarding the need for innovative antibiotics, FDAAA extended the duration of "market exclusivity" for new drugs, including antibiotics that meet certain criteria. Specifically, FDAAA extended the period of time that the sponsor of a drug meeting the criteria has exclusive rights to market the drug. In addition, FDAAA directed FDA to convene a public meeting to discuss the circumstances under which infectious diseases may qualify for grants or other incentives that may promote innovation, such as those offered by the Orphan Drug Act.[6]

FDAAA directed us to report on the impact of these provisions on new drugs. This report (1) assesses FDA's efforts to implement the FDAAA provision to help preserve antibiotic effectiveness by ensuring that breakpoints on labels are up to date and (2) examines the impact of the FDAAA provisions related to antibiotic innovation.

To examine FDA's efforts to implement the FDAAA provision related to antibiotic effectiveness by ensuring that breakpoints on labels are up to date, we obtained information on FDA's efforts to contact antibiotic sponsors regarding the accuracy of their antibiotics' labels, including their breakpoints.[7] Specifically, we examined information related to 210 antibiotics identified by FDA as those for which sponsors were responsible for evaluating and maintaining and, if necessary, updating the antibiotics' breakpoints on their labels. To assess the reliability of the information FDA used to identify these 210 antibiotics, we reviewed agency publications and related documentation, examined these data for

---

[6]See 21 U.S.C. §§ 360aa-360ee. The Orphan Drug Act provides incentives for the development of products that treat rare conditions affecting fewer than 200,000 people in the United States, including extended market exclusivity and grants to public and private entities and individuals to defray the costs of development.

[7]Breakpoints have been established for systemic antibiotics, which are administered intravenously, orally, or intramuscularly and affect the entire body. However, they have not been established for topical ant biotics, which are medicines applied to a localized area on the skin. In discussing breakpoints in this report, we use the term antibiotics to refer to systemic antibiotics for human use.

consistency, and interviewed knowledgeable agency officials. Through this review, we determined that FDA's information was incomplete. However, we found these data sufficiently reliable for our purposes. Of the 210 antibiotics, 126 were brand-name antibiotics and 84 were generic antibiotics—copies of brand-name drugs.[8] We contacted each of the 39 sponsors associated with the 210 antibiotics to obtain their views on FDA's actions in response to the FDAAA provision on antibiotic effectiveness.[9] We received written or oral comments from 26 of the 39 sponsors, representing 176 of the 210 antibiotics. (See app. I for a list of the 39 sponsors.) We discussed with FDA officials their plans to make up-to-date breakpoints on labels publicly available. We also reviewed FDA's guidance to drug manufacturers on maintaining up-to-date breakpoints on labels.

To examine the impact of the provisions contained in FDAAA related to antibiotic innovation, we determined whether drug sponsors had indicated an interest in the extended duration of market exclusivity for certain drugs, as specified in the law. We did this by determining whether sponsors (1) had been granted this extended market exclusivity for a new drug or (2) had submitted inquiries to FDA about this exclusivity. For context, we obtained data from FDA to determine the number of innovative antibiotics that had been developed both prior to and after the enactment of FDAAA. Specifically, we obtained data on all approvals for antibiotics containing new molecular entities (NME) for a 10-year period

---

[8]When a new drug is developed it is classified by its chemical type and therapeutic potential. Once FDA approves a new drug, it is marketed under a brand name—a proprietary, trademark-protected name—by a single sponsor. Only that original sponsor may use the brand name. A generic drug uses a name reflecting its chemical makeup and must be the same as the original drug in dosage form, strength, route of administration, and conditions of use. When a sponsor submits an application to FDA to bring a generic version onto the market, it must provide evidence that the generic drug is bioequivalent—a drug containing identical amounts of the same active ingredient(s) as the brand-name drug. There may be more than one sponsor marketing a generic version of the same brand-name drug.

[9]In most cases we attempted to contact the sponsor FDA identified. However, in some cases, such as when the original sponsor had since merged with another sponsor, been divested of its assets, or gone bankrupt, we contacted the subsequent sponsor. After performing these adjustments, we found that the 126 brand-name antibiotics were associated with 29 drug sponsors and the 84 generic antibiotics were associated with 23 drug sponsors. Thirteen of the sponsors marketed both brand-name and generic antibiotics among the 210 identified by FDA, so we contacted a total of 39 sponsors; 26 agreed to speak to us or to provide us with written or oral comments.

(2001-2010).[10] We also reviewed FDA's efforts related to the FDAAA requirement that it hold a public meeting to discuss incentives that may promote antibiotic innovation, and we examined the transcript of this meeting. We discussed with FDA whether drug sponsors had indicated an interest in marketing a new antibiotic under the provisions of the Orphan Drug Act. In addition, we reviewed FDA's policies and guidance regarding the application of existing incentives to antibiotics, including those found in the Orphan Drug Act, and obtained data on all approvals for antibiotics that received an orphan drug designation from 2001 through 2010. We asked the 26 antibiotic sponsors described above if incentives found in the FDAAA provision extending the period of exclusivity for certain drugs or the possible applicability of the Orphan Drug Act to antibiotics had or may affect their decisions to market, seek approval, or develop antibiotics. We also asked these sponsors to describe the incentives that would motivate them to develop and market antibiotics.

For both objectives, we reviewed FDA documents and interviewed FDA officials. In addition, to obtain stakeholder views on FDA's implementation of the relevant FDAAA provisions, we interviewed representatives from the Infectious Diseases Society of America, the Pharmaceutical Research and Manufacturers of America, the Generic Pharmaceutical Association, and the Clinical and Laboratory Standards Institute.

We conducted this performance audit from December 2010 to January 2012 in accordance with generally accepted government auditing standards. Those standards require that we plan and perform the audit to obtain sufficient, appropriate evidence to provide a reasonable basis for our findings and conclusions based on our audit objectives. We believe that the evidence obtained provides a reasonable basis for our findings and conclusions based on our audit objectives.

Background

FDA's mission is to protect the public health by ensuring the safety and effectiveness of human drugs marketed in the United States. The agency's responsibilities begin years before a drug is marketed and continue after a drug's approval.

---

[10]An NME is a drug that contains an active chemical substance that has never been approved for marketing in the United States in any form and is therefore generally considered innovative.

FDA and the Drug Approval Process

FDA oversees the drug development process. Among other things, FDA reviews drug sponsors' proposals for conducting clinical trials, assesses drug sponsors' applications for the approval of new drugs, and publishes guidance for industry on various topics. Once drugs are marketed in the United States, FDA has the responsibility to continue to monitor their safety and efficacy and to enforce drug sponsors' compliance with applicable laws and regulations. FDA also annually publishes a list of drugs approved for sale within the United States, the *Approved Drug Products with Therapeutic Equivalence Evaluations*, also known as the Orange Book. In addition, since February 2005, FDA has provided updates via the Electronic Orange Book on brand-name drug approvals the month they are approved and on generic drug approvals daily.[11]

FDA's Center for Drug Evaluation and Research is responsible for ensuring the safety and efficacy of drugs. Within this center, the Office of New Drugs is responsible for reviewing new drug applications (NDA), while the Office of Generic Drugs is responsible for reviewing applications for generic drugs, which are abbreviated new drug applications (ANDA).[12] NDAs and ANDAs must be submitted by sponsors and approved by FDA before a new brand-name or generic drug can be marketed in the United States. As part of the approval process, FDA reviews proposed labeling for both brand-name and generic drugs; a drug cannot be marketed without an FDA-approved label. Among other things, a drug's label contains information for health care providers and specifically cites the conditions and populations the drug has been approved to treat, as well as effective doses of the drug. Sponsors of both new brand-name and generic drugs are required to submit annual reports to FDA that include, for example, updates about the safety and effectiveness of their drugs; these annual reports are one way FDA monitors the safety and efficacy of drugs once they are available for sale.

---

[11]See http://www.accessdata.fda.gov/scripts/cder/ob/default.cfm.

[12]Manufacturers may submit an ANDA to FDA to seek approval to market a generic version of the drug after the period of exclusivity and any patents for a brand-name drug expire.

FDAAA Provisions Related to Antibiotic Effectiveness and Innovation

FDAAA contained three provisions related to antibiotic effectiveness and innovation, each of which required FDA to take certain actions. One provision required FDA to identify breakpoints "where such information is reasonably available," to periodically update them, and to make these up-to-date breakpoints publicly available within 30 days of identifying or updating them.[13]

A second provision extended the duration of market exclusivity from 3 years to 5 years for new drugs that meet certain detailed, scientific criteria.[14] Specifically, to obtain this additional exclusivity the NDA must be for a new drug consisting of a single enantiomer of a previously approved racemic drug.[15] The application for the drug must also be submitted for approval in a different therapeutic category than the previously approved drug and meet certain other requirements.[16] FDAAA specified that FDA use the therapeutic categories established by the United States Pharmacopeia to determine whether an application has been submitted for a separate therapeutic category than the previously approved drug.[17] It also required FDA to publish the list of therapeutic categories developed by this organization that were in effect on the date of the enactment of FDAAA.

A third provision authorized funding for grants and contracts under the Orphan Drug Act and required FDA to convene a public meeting to discuss incentives, such as those included in the Orphan Drug Act, to develop or otherwise obtain market exclusivity for antibiotics that treat

---

[13]Pub. L. No. 110-85, § 1111, 121 Stat. 823, 975-76 (2007).

[14]The provision applies to new drugs of any type that meet the criteria, not just antibiotics. Pub. L. No. 110-85, § 1113, 121 Stat. 823, 976-77 (2007).

[15]A racemic drug consists of two enantiomers—molecules that are identical in atomic constitution and bonding, but are mirror images of each other—in equal proportions. There may be therapeutic benefits from isolating a single enantiomer from a racemic drug.

[16]Other criteria necessary to qualify for this extended market exclusivity include a requirement that the sponsor must submit full reports of new clinical investigations and the application must not rely on any investigations that are part of the application submitted for the previously approved drug. The extended exclusivity is only available for applications submitted before October 1, 2012.

[17]The United States Pharmacopeia is a nongovernmental, official public standards-setting authority for prescription and over-the-counter drugs. It sets standards for the quality, purity, identity, and strength of these products. Its Model Guidelines is a list of therapeutic categories and pharmacologic classes.

serious and life-threatening infectious diseases.[18] Incentives are intended to counter some of the business risks a drug sponsor must undertake when developing antibiotics. For example, the Orphan Drug Act provides incentives including a 7-year period of marketing exclusivity to sponsors of approved orphan drugs, a tax credit of 50 percent of the cost of conducting human clinical testing, research grants for clinical testing of new therapies to treat orphan diseases, and exemption from the fees that are typically charged when sponsors submit NDAs for FDA's review. Sponsors may also be eligible for a faster review of their applications for market approval.

FDA's and Drug Sponsors' Responsibilities to Ensure Up-to-Date Breakpoints on Labels

Sponsors of all drugs are required to keep the information on their drug labels accurate. Unlike labels for most other types of drugs, labels for antibiotics contain breakpoints.[19] These breakpoints may continue to change over time, and the sponsors of antibiotics are tasked with the additional responsibility of maintaining up-to-date breakpoints on labels. Although sponsors are required to maintain up-to-date breakpoints on their labels, FDA has acknowledged that many antibiotics are labeled with outdated breakpoints. Outdated breakpoints can result in health care providers unknowingly selecting ineffective treatments, which can also contribute to additional bacterial resistance to antibiotics.

Monitoring breakpoints on labels and keeping them up to date can be a challenging process. The most accurate way to monitor and determine if a breakpoint on a label is up to date is to conduct both clinical trials and laboratory studies, but these can be difficult and expensive and may not be appropriate in all circumstances. For example, clinical trials require the enrollment of large numbers of patients, which may be difficult to achieve, to ensure an understanding of a drug's safety and effectiveness against specific bacteria. Enrollment may also be difficult for clinical trials involving antibiotic-resistant bacteria. Unlike clinical trials for a new cancer drug, for example, where researchers are able to target drugs to a patient population with a specific type of cancer, this may not necessarily

---

[18]Pub. L. No. 110-85, § 1112, 121 Stat. 823, 976 (2007).

[19]See 21 C.F.R. § 201.57(c)(2)(i)(C) (2011). In general, breakpoints are established based on in vivo and in vitro information provided by the sponsor. In vivo testing is that which is performed in a living organism, such as an animal, while in vitro testing is performed in a laboratory using components of a living organism.

be the case for antibacterial drugs. There are no rapid diagnostic tests available to help a researcher identify patients with antibiotic-resistant infections who would be eligible for such trials. Laboratory studies, such as susceptibility testing, can be less costly than clinical trials; however, they still require significant microbiology expertise. Susceptibility testing reveals an antibiotic's breakpoint—that is, its ability to kill or inhibit the growth of a specific bacterial pathogen. As such, the results of such tests can provide a sponsor with some data to help update its antibiotic label with more accurate information. Guidelines for developing appropriate susceptibility tests are available from standards-setting organizations, such as the Clinical and Laboratory Standards Institute.[20] Sponsors may obtain information from such organizations to help them conduct susceptibility tests for their antibiotics or otherwise determine if the breakpoints on their antibiotic labels are up to date. According to FDA officials, much of this information is available free online and at conferences.[21]

When new information becomes available that may cause the label to become inaccurate, false, or misleading—such as information on increased bacterial resistance to antibiotics—drug sponsors are responsible for updating their drug labels.[22] Label changes of this type require FDA's approval.[23] A sponsor must submit an application supplement to FDA with evidence to support the need for a label change. A sponsor's responsibility for maintaining a drug's label persists throughout the life cycle of the drug—that is, from the time the drug is first approved until FDA withdraws its approval of the drug.[24] A drug is not

---

[20]The Clinical and Laboratory Standards Institute is a consensus-based organization that develops standards with input from stakeholders in government, industry, and laboratories to promote accurate antimicrobial susceptibility testing and appropriate reporting.

[21]For example, FDA told us that scientific information is discussed twice yearly at the Clinical and Laboratory Standards Institute meetings and may be available to interested persons by request or online at its website (http://www.clsi.org).

[22]See 21 C.F.R. § 201.56(a)(2) (2011).

[23]See 21 C.F.R. §§ 314.70, 314.97 (2011).

[24]The process to withdraw approval of a drug can be initiated by either FDA or the drug sponsor, for a variety of reasons (e.g., if the drug poses an imminent hazard to public health, if there are other safety concerns, or if there are concerns about the drug's effectiveness in dosage or strength) or if the sponsor makes a business decision to no longer manufacture the drug. See 21 C.F.R. § 314.150 (2011).

considered withdrawn until FDA publishes a *Federal Register* notice officially announcing its withdrawal. A sponsor may also decide to discontinue manufacturing a drug without withdrawal. Sponsors that decide to discontinue marketing a drug are still responsible for maintaining accurate labels. Unlike a drug that is withdrawn, a discontinued drug for which approval has not been withdrawn is one that the sponsor has stopped marketing, but that it may resume marketing without obtaining permission to do so from FDA. Discontinued drugs are identified as such in the discontinued section of the Orange Book.[25]

FDA designates certain drugs as "reference-listed drugs" and the sponsors of these drugs play an important role in ensuring the accuracy of drug labels, especially for antibiotic labels. A reference-listed drug is an approved drug product to which generic versions are compared. FDA assigns at least one marketed drug per active ingredient, dosage, and route of administration as a reference-listed drug and indicates this status in the Orange Book. FDA generally designates brand-name drugs—those approved through the NDA process—as reference-listed drugs at the time of their approval. Sponsors of generic drugs—those approved through the ANDA process—must cite or "reference" the reference-listed drug in their applications. Sponsors of ANDAs must demonstrate that their generic drugs are bioequivalent to, and perform in the same manner as, the reference-listed drug. In addition, sponsors of generic drugs are required to follow the labels of the corresponding reference-listed drug.[26] They therefore are expected to incorporate any updates made to the label of the reference-listed drug, such as new safety warnings, indications, or up-

---

[25]FDA does not have a standard mechanism for determining whether a company has actually discontinued marketing a drug. Agency officials stated that they most often become aware of a discontinued drug when they review sponsors' annual reports or when a generic sponsor contacts FDA and informs the agency that an approved drug included in the Orange Book no longer appears to be marketed, and thus cannot be referenced in the generic sponsor's ANDA as the product it intends to copy. The officials added that there is no specific amount of time that must pass before a nonmarketed drug becomes listed as discontinued.

[26]Federal regulations allow ANDA's labels to differ from the label of the corresponding reference-listed drug in certain ways, such as manufacturer name or expiration date. See 21 C.F.R. § 314.94(a)(8)(iv) (2011).

to-date breakpoints, into their generic drugs' labels.[27] A drug maintains its reference-listed drug designation until its approval is withdrawn or a finding is made by FDA that a discontinued reference-listed drug was withdrawn from the market for safety or effectiveness reasons.[28] In either of these cases, FDA will designate a different drug as the reference-listed drug and publish this change in the Orange Book. FDA will generally designate the generic version of the drug with the largest market share as the new reference-listed drug. In this case, the labels of other generic versions of the drug will be expected to follow the label of the newly designated generic, reference-listed drug.

FDA Has Not Taken Sufficient Steps to Ensure That Antibiotic Labels Contain Up-to-Date Information

FDA has not taken sufficient steps to implement the FDAAA provision regarding preserving antibiotic effectiveness by ensuring that antibiotic labels contain up-to-date breakpoints. In 2008 FDA requested that sponsors respond to the agency regarding whether their antibiotics' labels included up-to-date breakpoints, but FDA has not yet confirmed whether the majority of these labels are accurate. FDA also took the step of issuing guidance in 2009 on sponsors' responsibility to maintain up-to-date breakpoints on their antibiotics' labels, but the agency has not been systematically tracking sponsors' responsiveness.

---

[27]A case decided by the U.S. Supreme Court, *Pliva, Inc. v. Mensing*, addressed the obligations of generic drug sponsors to keep their drug labels up to date. The Supreme Court ruled on June 23, 2011, that such sponsors cannot be held liable under state law for failing to include new safety warnings on their labels because warnings need to be identical to those on the label of the corresponding reference-listed drug. The court ruled that it is impossible for sponsors to comply with both federal law prohibiting generic drug sponsors from changing their labels from that of the reference-listed drug without FDA's permission and state law requiring sponsors to update their labels when they learn of new safety information, and that generic manufacturers must comply with the federal requirement. See Pliva, Inc. v. Mensing, 131 S.Ct. 2567 (2011). FDA is in the process of reviewing the court's decision and determining what impact it may have on generic drug sponsors and sponsors of reference-listed drugs and what action FDA should take.

[28]See 21 C.F.R. § 314.161(e) 2011.

FDA Has Taken Some Steps, but Has Not Yet Confirmed That Breakpoint Information Is Up-to-Date for Many Antibiotics

Although FDA has taken steps to update breakpoint information on antibiotic labels, as of November 2011, it has not confirmed that the information is up to date for most reference-listed antibiotics. As one step in FDA's efforts to implement the FDAAA provision regarding antibiotic effectiveness, FDA identified 210 antibiotics and, in January and February 2008, sent letters to the sponsors of these drugs reminding them of the importance of regularly updating the breakpoints on their antibiotic labels. In addition, the letters requested that sponsors evaluate and maintain the currency of breakpoints included on their labels and within 30 days submit evidence to FDA showing that the breakpoints were either current or needed revision. Sponsors that could not submit this evidence within 30 days were advised to provide the agency with a timetable for when they expected to respond with this information. If sponsors determined that their antibiotic labels needed revision, the agency's letter instructed them to submit a label supplement. FDA's letters also highlighted to sponsors that all subsequent annual reports should include an evaluation of these breakpoints and document the status of any needed changes to the antibiotic label.

As of November 2011, over 3.5 years after FDA sent its letters, 146, or 70 percent, of the 210 antibiotics are still labeled with breakpoints that have not been updated or confirmed to be up to date. For 78 of the 146 antibiotics, FDA has not yet received a submission regarding the currency of the breakpoints; for 12 of the antibiotics, the sponsors' submissions are pending FDA review; and for 56 of the antibiotics, FDA determined that the sponsors' submission was inaccurate or incomplete and therefore requested a revision or additional information. Thus far, FDA has determined that 64, or 30 percent, of the 210 antibiotics have up-to-date breakpoints (see fig. 1). (See app. II for more details on the status of the labels of the 210 antibiotics.)

Figure 1: Status of Labels for 210 Antibiotics

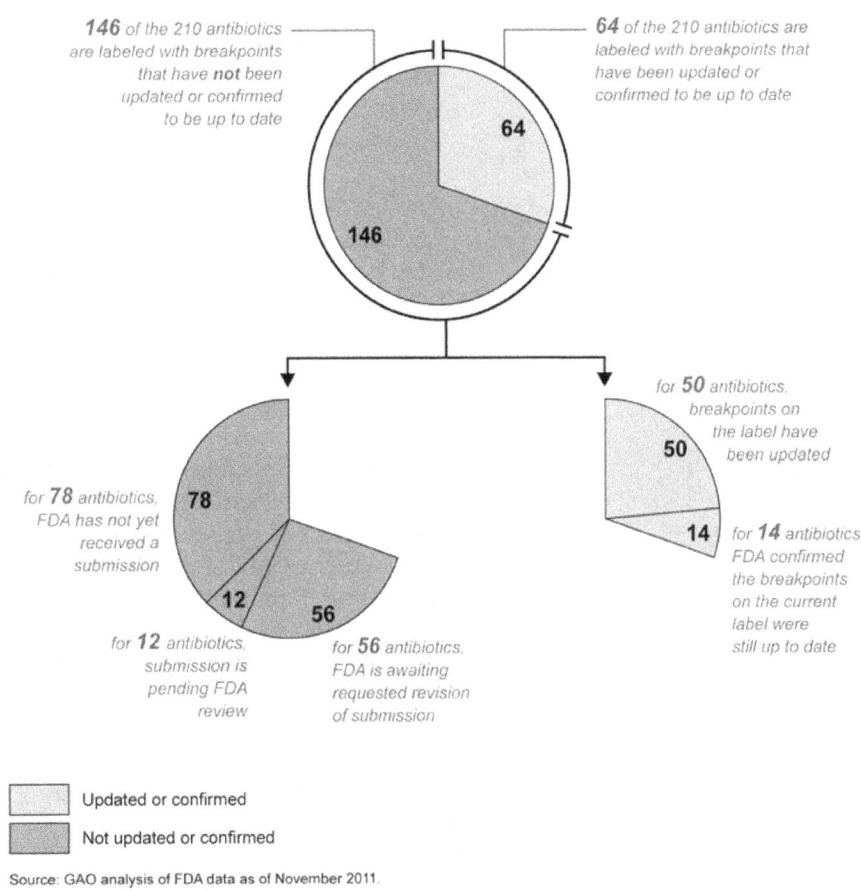

146 of the 210 antibiotics are labeled with breakpoints that have **not** been updated or confirmed to be up to date

64 of the 210 antibiotics are labeled with breakpoints that have been updated or confirmed to be up to date

for 78 antibiotics, FDA has not yet received a submission

for 12 antibiotics, submission is pending FDA review

for 56 antibiotics, FDA is awaiting requested revision of submission

for 50 antibiotics, breakpoints on the label have been updated

for 14 antibiotics, FDA confirmed the breakpoints on the current label were still up to date

☐ Updated or confirmed

☐ Not updated or confirmed

Source: GAO analysis of FDA data as of November 2011.

One reason so many antibiotics still have breakpoints that FDA has not confirmed to be up to date is that many sponsors have not fulfilled the responsibilities outlined in FDA's 2008 letters. FDA officials stated that the agency has followed up with sponsors that had not responded at all to the 2008 letters; however, it did not begin to do so until 2010—2 years after it asked sponsors to respond within 30 days—and two sponsors have still not informed FDA when they intend to submit the requested information. FDA officials told us that they routinely monitor the status of all requested submissions that they have not yet received. In particular, they told us that they have contacted sponsors to set time frames for submitting the requested information, and that they follow up with sponsors that do not submit information within the time frames established. FDA has not pursued regulatory action against any of these sponsors. FDA officials stated that the agency could take regulatory action against a sponsor whose label contained outdated breakpoints, as federal regulations require all sponsors of drugs to maintain accurate labels. However, the officials added that in order for FDA to take regulatory action against a sponsor, FDA would first have to be able to prove that the breakpoint on the antibiotic label was not up to date.

Another reason many antibiotics still have breakpoints on their labels that FDA has not confirmed to be up to date is that FDA faced difficulty in keeping up with the workload that resulted from sponsors' breakpoint submissions. According to FDA officials, it should take 1 to 3 months for the agency to review such submissions when staff are available and the submissions include all of the necessary information. However, it took FDA longer than a year to review many of the submissions it received, and as of November 2011, FDA still had a backlog of five submissions from 2008. FDA officials identified four factors that have contributed to the lengthy time between when the agency received a submission and when it completed its review. First, FDA officials explained that the submissions sent in response to the agency's 2008 letter generated a larger number of supplements than normal, adding significantly to FDA's existing workload of label supplements. Second, some of the submissions required significantly more resources to review than typical label supplements, because of challenging scientific issues or difficulties obtaining data. Third, some of the sponsors' submissions were inaccurate or did not include all necessary information. Fourth, FDA staff spent a significant amount of time answering questions from sponsors, tracking responses, and following up when needed.

Some of the sponsors we obtained comments from expressed frustration at how long it took FDA to review their submissions, especially given that bacterial resistance to antibiotics is not static and breakpoints may continue to change over time.[29] Specifically, 3 of the 26 sponsors we obtained comments from stated that they are concerned that the

---

[29]When asked how the FDAAA provision on antibiotic effectiveness influenced their interest in developing, seeking FDA approval to market, or continuing to market antibiotics, officials from all sponsors that replied to this question told us that it did not have an influence. However, eight sponsors noted that the financial burdens associated with maintaining up-to-date breakpoints could deter a sponsor from marketing an antibiotic.

breakpoints they submitted may be outdated by the time FDA completes its review. One of these sponsors told us that it was advised by FDA to refrain from submitting new information before the agency completed its review of the sponsor's previously submitted label supplement. According to the sponsor, FDA officials said that providing new information would result in the sponsor's submission going to the end of FDA's review queue.

While the fact that breakpoints on the labels of 146 antibiotics may not be up to date is troubling, there are additional reasons for concern. First, nearly all of these 146 antibiotics are reference-listed drugs—thus, in addition to the labels of these drugs, the labels of the generic antibiotics that follow the labels of the reference-listed antibiotics are also uncertain. Second, because bacterial resistance to antibiotics is not static, some of the breakpoints for the 64 antibiotics that FDA has confirmed through its review as up to date may have since become out of date. Third, FDA's list of 210 drugs did not include a complete list of all the antibiotics for which sponsors are responsible for evaluating and maintaining the breakpoints on their labels. For example, FDA did not include any brand-name drugs that were discontinued at the time the agency compiled its list, and also did not include some antibiotics that were reference-listed drugs at that time.[30] FDA officials were unsure how many antibiotics were omitted, but estimated that the number was low. Given the uncertainty surrounding the 146 antibiotics whose breakpoints have not yet been confirmed as well as the antibiotics omitted from FDA's 2008 request to sponsors, more than two-thirds of reference-listed antibiotic labels may contain out-of-date breakpoints.

FDA Issued Guidance on Sponsors' Responsibility to Evaluate and Maintain Up-to-Date Breakpoints, but Has Not Been Tracking Their Responses

Another step FDA took to implement the FDAAA provision regarding preserving the effectiveness of antibiotics was to issue guidance that reminded sponsors of the requirement to maintain accurate labels, and thus, their responsibility to keep information about breakpoints up to date.[31] FDA officials stated that in part because the agency received questions in response to its 2008 letters, officials determined that it would be useful to issue guidance. FDA first issued draft guidance in June 2008

---

[30]Sponsors of discontinued, brand-name antibiotics retain responsibility for evaluating and maintaining the breakpoints on their labels.

[31]See 21 C.F.R. § 201.56(a)(2) (2011).

and finalized it a year later, in June 2009. The guidance specified that the sponsors of brand-name and generic antibiotics that are designated as reference-listed drugs are responsible for evaluating their breakpoints on labels at least annually and should include this evaluation in the sponsor's annual report to FDA.[32] When we asked for clarification as to whether the guidance language limited this responsibility to the sponsors of those brand-name antibiotics that are reference listed, FDA officials told us that the guidance applied to sponsors of all brand-name antibiotics—both those that were and were not reference listed, including those that are discontinued—as well as sponsors of reference-listed, generic antibiotics. The guidance also described approaches sponsors could take to determine up-to-date breakpoints for their antibiotics. While FDA's 2008 letters to certain sponsors communicated much of the same information, FDA's guidance was the first time that FDA specified (1) which sponsors are responsible for evaluating their breakpoints, including that this responsibility applied to sponsors of generic, reference-listed antibiotics, and (2) the frequency with which sponsors needed to perform these evaluations.

FDA has not been systematically tracking whether sponsors have been responsive to the guidance. Specifically, FDA does not know what percentage of antibiotic annual reports have included an evaluation of breakpoints. At our request, FDA reviewed a small sample of annual reports and this review suggested that sponsors' responsiveness to the annual reporting responsibility is low. FDA reviewed the most recent annual reports for 19 of the 64 antibiotics that FDA confirmed to be labeled with up-to-date breakpoints after receiving a response to the agency's 2008 letters. FDA found that 10 of the 19, or just over half, of these annual reports included an evaluation of the antibiotics' breakpoints.[33] Given the low level of sponsors' responsiveness for this group of antibiotics—that is, those for which a sponsor already responded to FDA's 2008 letter with a submission regarding the currency of their breakpoints—the overall rate for all antibiotics is likely even lower.

---

[32]See FDA, *Guidance for Industry: Updating Labeling for Susceptibility Test Information in Systemic Antibacterial Drug Products and Antimicrobial Susceptibility Testing Devices* (June 2009).

[33]FDA looked at a subset of the 64 antibiotics that were also brand-name drugs and for which the sponsor had submitted its most recent annual report electronically. Three of the 19 antibiotics in FDA's sample had annual reports that noted that a label supplement was recently approved but had not been implemented in time to be reflected in the report.

Because bacterial resistance to antibiotics is not static, sponsors that do not follow the guidance by evaluating their breakpoints on a regular basis and sharing the results of their evaluation with FDA are unlikely to be able to maintain accurate labels. FDA officials stated that they plan to track compliance with the guidance in one of the agency's drug databases by January 1, 2012. FDA plans to have all annual reports for antibiotics reviewed by FDA microbiologists who will use a standardized form to document the assessment of the antibiotics' breakpoints. In addition, the agency plans to track whether the annual report included an evaluation of the antibiotics' breakpoints in an FDA database. FDA plans to follow up with sponsors that do not include a complete evaluation of antibiotic breakpoints in their annual reports to inform them about what information was missing.

Some sponsors, particularly sponsors of generic, reference-listed antibiotics, may not be following FDA's guidance because they are confused as to whether the responsibility to evaluate and maintain up-to-date breakpoints on their labels, as described in the guidance, applies to them. Fifteen sponsors we obtained comments from manufactured at least one generic, reference-listed antibiotic—all were responsible for evaluating and maintaining their breakpoints. Of these 15, 7 sponsors expressed some form of confusion regarding their responsibility.[34] Five of these 7 sponsors stated that their strategy for ensuring that the breakpoints on their generic antibiotic labels were up to date was to follow the breakpoints on the label of the corresponding brand-name drug. Two of the 5 were even more specific and added that their generic antibiotics were only designated reference-listed drugs "by default" and that their strategy was to follow the label of the brand-name drug—even if the brand-name drug was discontinued. One other sponsor was unsure whether any of its generic antibiotics were reference-listed drugs or what implications such a designation would have. A seventh sponsor understood the responsibilities associated with having a generic antibiotic that was designated a reference-listed drug, but was under the impression that its generic antibiotic was not a reference-listed drug.

---

[34]Cumulatively, as of early 2008, these sponsors manufactured 35 generic, reference-listed antibiotics.

FDA officials told us that it is a sponsor's responsibility to routinely monitor FDA's Orange Book to determine if any of its drugs become designated a reference-listed drug. However, FDA's June 2009 guidance is silent on sponsors' responsibility to consistently monitor the Orange Book to determine if one of their drugs has become, or ceases to be, a reference-listed drug. The officials acknowledged that there is no process or mechanism for notifying sponsors when one of their drugs becomes, or is no longer, a reference-listed drug. The guidance was also not explicit about FDA's view that the responsibility described in the guidance also applied to sponsors of discontinued brand-name antibiotics.

The guidance also explained that FDA intended to comply with FDAAA's requirement that it identify, periodically update, and make publicly available up-to-date breakpoints by using two approaches. First, the guidance explained that the agency would review breakpoints referenced in the labeling of individual drug products and post any approved labels on the Internet.[35] FDA officials told us that this is the approach FDA has thus far used to make up-to-date breakpoints publicly available.[36] Second, FDA's guidance also stated that it would, when appropriate, recognize standards used to determine breakpoints from one or more standards-setting organizations and publish these in the *Federal Register*.[37] FDA has not yet used this approach and did not mention a specific plan or timetable to do so. FDA officials told us that publishing this information in the *Federal Register* could make the review process quicker as sponsors would then have ready access to standards already recognized by FDA.

---

[35]FDA specified that it would publish labels with up-to-date breakpoints on the Drugs@FDA (*http://www.accessdata.fda.gov/scripts/cder/drugsatfda*) or DailyMed (*http://dailymed.nlm.nih.gov/dailymed/about.cfm*) websites.

[36]In October 2011, FDA notified us that it had also begun posting on a separate website a list of all the antibiotic labels it has reviewed since 2008, along with the date on which FDA determined the breakpoints on each label to be current. This list includes both antibiotics for which FDA approved a label supplement and those for which FDA determined the breakpoints on the current label were up to date. See http://www.fda.gov/AboutFDA/CentersOffices/OfficeofMedicalProductsandTobacco/CDER/ucm275763.htm.

[37]The guidance also contained information on how sponsors should respond to the publication of a recognized standard in the *Federal Register*. According to the guidance, sponsors of brand-name antibiotics and generic, reference-listed antibiotics would have 90 days from FDA's publication of a standard to submit updated product labeling, including breakpoints based on the newly recognized standard, or provide a written explanation of why the recognized standard was not applicable to their antibiotics.

For example, publishing this information may be helpful for some sponsors, such as those that do not have the microbiology expertise to update their own breakpoints. While FDA officials said that they have been making updated breakpoints publicly available, the agency's guidance regarding these alternative approaches may be causing confusion among some sponsors that are anticipating the publication of breakpoints from standards-setting organizations in the *Federal Register*. This was the case for one sponsor we obtained comments from, which stopped purchasing data from a standard-setting organization because it believed FDA would be publishing recognized standards in the *Federal Register*.

FDAAA Provisions Related to Innovation Do Not Appear to Have Encouraged the Development of New Antibiotics

The FDAAA provision that grants extended market exclusivity has not resulted in any sponsors submitting NDAs for antibiotics that qualify for this exclusivity. Additionally, as required by FDAAA, FDA held a public meeting to discuss incentives, such as those available under the Orphan Drug Act, to encourage antibiotic innovation. However, no changes were made to the availability of current incentives nor were any new incentives established following the public meeting.

No New Drug Applications for Antibiotics Have Been Submitted under FDAAA's Extended Market Exclusivity Provision

To date, drug sponsors, including those we received comments from, have not submitted any NDAs for antibiotics as a result of the FDAAA provision granting additional market exclusivity for new drugs containing single enantiomers of previously approved racemic drugs. According to FDA officials, they have received very few inquiries regarding this provision and as of November 2011, no NDAs for antibiotics have been submitted that would qualify for this exclusivity. FDA officials noted that because it is a narrowly targeted provision, they are unsure if any existing racemic drug could qualify. None of the drug sponsors from which we obtained comments said that this FDAAA provision provided a sufficient incentive to develop a new antibiotic of this type.[38]

FDA officials stated that it was unlikely that this provision would have an impact on antibiotic innovation. The officials stated that the requirement that the single enantiomer of the approved drug be in a separate

---

[38]One of the 26 drug sponsors we obtained information from did not provide a response to our questions on the FDAAA provision related to antibiotic innovation.

therapeutic category would be challenging for antibiotic sponsors to meet. The officials noted that this market exclusivity was not limited to antibiotics. One drug sponsor we spoke with stated that it is pursuing this market exclusivity for a drug that is not an antibiotic.

The lack of NDAs for antibiotics submitted in response to this FDAAA provision is consistent with the overall trend in the approval of innovative antibiotic NDAs. The number of annual approvals of antibiotic NMEs from 2001 through 2010 has not changed significantly since the passage of FDAAA. Specifically, the annual number of antibiotic NME approvals was two or less for the years prior to, and one or less for the years following, the enactment of FDAAA. Because drug development is a lengthy process—sponsors spend, on average, 15 years developing a new drug—it may be too early to ascertain the full impact of FDAAA on antibiotic innovation. However, the extended exclusivity provided for in FDAAA is only available to sponsors submitting qualifying NDAs before October 1, 2012.

FDA Public Meeting Required by FDAAA Facilitated Discussion of Existing and Potential Incentives for Antibiotic Innovation

As required by FDAAA, FDA held a public meeting on April 28, 2008, to explore whether and how existing incentives and potential new incentives could be applied to promote the development of antibiotics as well as to discuss whether infectious diseases may qualify for grants or other incentives that may promote innovation. The meeting provided an opportunity to gather input from stakeholders and address their concerns. However, although potential new incentives and changes to current ones were suggested at the meeting, many of these suggestions—such as tax incentives and extended market exclusivities—would require a statutory change.

One of the discussion topics at the public meeting related to the circumstances under which antibiotics could qualify for incentives provided under the Orphan Drug Act, which is intended to stimulate the development of drugs for rare diseases—conditions that affect fewer than 200,000 people in the United States. Following the public meeting, FDA responded in writing to an inquiry from one stakeholder to clarify that an antibiotic could qualify for an orphan drug designation when the drug's use is restricted to the treatment of a small population of patients with an infection caused by a specific pathogen. Our examination of FDA data suggests that orphan drug designation is not common for antibiotics. These data show that the annual number of antibiotics that received an orphan drug designation from 2001 to 2007—when FDAAA was enacted—was three drugs or fewer each year. The number of antibiotics that received orphan drug designation following FDAAA's enactment in 2007 has remained constant at this rate through 2010. Additionally, not all antibiotics that have been awarded orphan drug designation have been or will apply to be approved for marketing. Of the 15 antibiotics that received an orphan drug designation from 2001 through 2010, only 1 was approved for marketing as of November 2011.[39]

In addition to discussing the applicability of the Orphan Drug Act, the agency gathered input during the public meeting from drug sponsors and other parties—such as those in academia and professional associations—on serious and life-threatening infectious diseases, antibiotic resistance, and incentives for antibiotic innovation. The incentives mentioned as useful mechanisms to encourage the innovation and marketing of antibiotics were both financial and regulatory in nature and are summarized in table 1.

Table 1: Incentives Discussed at 2008 FDA Public Meeting to Promote Antibiotic Innovation

- Tax incentives for research and development
- Federal funding for certain early research activities
- Intellectual property incentives, such as extended market exclusivity
- Fast track approval process—a process designed to facilitate the innovation of and expedite FDA's review of drugs that treat serious diseases and fill an unmet need
- Priority review voucher for quicker FDA review of a future drug application
- Regulatory clarity during the drug approval process, such as clearer guidelines for conducting clinical trials
- Placing antibiotics in a separate regulatory category so that sponsors may receive unique economic benefits, such as extended market exclusivities or tax benefits

Source: GAO analysis of the transcript of FDA's public meeting held on April 28, 2008.

Consistent with the types of incentives identified by the participants at FDA's public meeting, sponsors that we obtained comments from mentioned multiple incentives. They suggested that a combination of both financial and regulatory incentives may prompt sponsors to develop new antibiotics. These comments were consistent with the findings presented

---

[39]This antibiotic—Inhalational Aztreonam—provides inhalation therapy for the control of gram-negative bacteria in the respiratory tract of patients with cystic fibrosis. It was granted orphan drug designation before the enactment of FDAAA, on March 12, 2002, and was approved for marketing on February 22, 2010.

in a 2009 study on antibiotic innovation.[40] When we asked these 26 drug sponsors to identify the incentives that would encourage them to develop antibiotics, market exclusivities were the most frequently identified incentive to develop antibiotics, mentioned by half (13 of 26) of the sponsors. Six drug sponsors noted that regulatory clarity, including specific guidance, would be an incentive to promote the innovation of antibiotics. Three drug sponsors also stated that priority review vouchers for new antibiotics—similar to those FDAAA made available to certain sponsors that received approval of treatments for tropical diseases—would promote antibiotic innovation because they could allow a future antibiotic to reach the market faster. For NDAs, FDA's goal for priority review is to make a decision regarding drug approvals on 90 percent of the applications within 6 months of their submission. However, when considering incentives to promote antibiotic innovation, it is important to note that any incentive that extends market exclusivity for an innovator of antibiotics will, by definition, delay the entry of generic versions of those antibiotics into the market.[41] (App. III contains a timeline of FDA's actions to implement FDAAA provisions related to antibiotic effectiveness and innovation.)

Conclusions

The growing public health threat associated with bacterial resistance to antibiotics makes the development of new antibiotics critical. Although FDAAA contained a provision to encourage the development of certain antibiotics, no sponsor has submitted an application for a new drug that meets the law's specific criteria. FDAAA also recognized that up-to-date breakpoints are vital to preserving the effectiveness of antibiotics. Antibiotic labels containing out-of-date breakpoints can lead clinicians to choose less effective treatments and provide additional opportunities for bacteria to develop resistance. Out-of-date breakpoints on labels of reference-listed antibiotics also have a ripple effect on the accuracy of the labels of other antibiotics because other sponsors must match the labels

---

[40]London School of Economics and Political Science, *Policies and Incentives for Promoting Innovation in Antibiotic Research* (London: 2009).

[41]As members of the Interagency Task Force on Antimicrobial Resistance, which includes a variety of other federal agencies, HHS and FDA are involved in additional efforts to encourage the development of new antibiotics. For example, HHS is currently sponsoring a study to evaluate incentives to promote the development of antibacterial drugs for human use as well as rapid diagnostic tests. A report describing the study results is expected to be issued in 2012.

of the corresponding reference-listed drugs. However, more than 4 years after FDAAA's enactment, there continues to be uncertainty about the accuracy of the labels of more than two thirds of reference-listed antibiotics, as well as those of the generic antibiotics that are required to follow these drugs' labels.

The steps FDA has taken since the enactment of FDAAA have been insufficient to ensure that all antibiotics have up-to-date breakpoints on their labels. The agency has acted with neither decisiveness nor a sense of urgency. First, FDA has not yet completed reviewing the submissions it received in response to its 2008 request and many sponsors still have not provided FDA with needed information. Further, FDA officials told us that they sent letters to sponsors of 210 antibiotics. These sponsors were responsible for evaluating and maintaining, and if necessary, updating the breakpoints on their labels; however, FDA's request was not made to all the antibiotic sponsors that held this responsibility. While the agency did follow up with sponsors, this was not done in a timely manner. FDA's review of sponsors' submissions has also been time-consuming; given that sponsors are expected to provide information on the effectiveness of these breakpoints annually. It is unclear how the agency plans to keep up with this workload if sponsors' fulfillment of this responsibility improves.

Second, FDA's issuance of guidance to specify the responsibilities of antibiotics' sponsors to evaluate breakpoints appears to have been unsuccessful at encouraging all sponsors to fulfill these responsibilities. The comments we received from drug sponsors indicate that some antibiotic sponsors remain confused about this responsibility—either because they did not know that their antibiotics were reference-listed drugs or because they interpreted the June 2009 FDA guidance differently than FDA intended. Without formal notification that their antibiotics have been designated as reference-listed drugs and a clarification of their responsibilities, sponsors may continue to be unaware of, or have differing interpretations of a responsibility that ultimately helps preserve antibiotic effectiveness.

The pace of FDA's actions—many of which remain incomplete—means that the majority of antibiotics we examined may have out-of-date breakpoints on their labels that could result in the prescription of ineffective treatments by health care providers and further contribute to antibiotic resistance. This requires concerted action on the part of the agency to help preserve the effectiveness of currently available antibiotics.

Recommendations for Executive Action

We recommend that the Commissioner of FDA take the following six actions to help ensure that antibiotics are accurately labeled:

- expeditiously review sponsors' submissions regarding the breakpoints on their antibiotics' labels;

- take steps to obtain breakpoint information from sponsors that have not yet submitted breakpoint information in response to the 2008 letters sent by the agency;

- ensure that all sponsors responsible for the annual review of breakpoints on their antibiotics' labels—including discontinued brand-name antibiotics and reference-listed antibiotics designated since 2008—have been reminded of their responsibility to evaluate and maintain up-to-date breakpoints;

- establish a process to track sponsors' submissions of breakpoint information included in their annual reports to ensure that such information is submitted to FDA and reviewed by the agency in a timely manner;

- notify sponsors when one of their drugs becomes or ceases to be a reference-listed drug; and

- clarify or provide new guidance on which antibiotic sponsors are responsible for annually evaluating and maintaining up-to-date breakpoints on drug labels.

Agency Comments and Our Evaluation

HHS reviewed a draft of this report and provided written comments, which are reprinted in appendix IV. In its comments, HHS acknowledged the importance of updating antibacterial breakpoints and said that FDA is committed to ensuring that breakpoint information on drug labels is up to date. Although HHS did not specifically indicate whether it agreed with our recommendations, the agency stated that it will consider all of them as it continues to improve its processes to ensure that antibacterial drug labels contain up-to-date breakpoint information. HHS also stated that FDA has already taken steps to expedite the review of sponsor submissions regarding updated breakpoint information, which is consistent with our recommendations.

In addition, HHS expressed concern that our report did not fully capture the challenges associated with updating the labels of antibacterial drugs. HHS summarized the approach FDA used to address the provision in FDAAA related to antibiotic effectiveness and highlighted the challenges sponsors face in obtaining currently relevant and adequate scientific data to assess antibiotic breakpoints. However, we believe that our report accurately describes the same actions that HHS outlined in its comments. Similarly, we believe that our report acknowledges the challenges surrounding sponsors' responsibility to maintain up-to-date breakpoints. We recognize that these challenges pose difficulties for both sponsors and FDA. However, FDA is ultimately responsible for ensuring that drugs, including antibiotics, are safe and effective. Despite the agency's efforts, 4 years have elapsed since FDA first began contacting drug sponsors regarding the accuracy of the breakpoints on 210 of their antibiotics' labels. Yet there continues to be uncertainty about the accuracy of the labels for two-thirds of these drugs. Given the serious threat to public health posed by antibiotic resistance, we believe that it is important that our recommendations are implemented, in order to help preserve the effectiveness of these critical drugs.

Finally, HHS provided us with new information, reporting that as of December 12, 2011, the labeling for 66 antibacterial drugs has been updated or found to be correct. This is an increase of 2 antibacterial drugs, up from the 64 antibacterial drugs that are cited in our report. We include this information here, but did not revise our report, as HHS did not provide a complete update regarding all of the 210 antibiotics discussed in this report. HHS also provided technical comments that were incorporated, as appropriate.

We are sending copies of this report to the Secretary of Health and Human Services and appropriate congressional committees. In addition, the report will be available at no charge on the GAO website at http://www.gao.gov.

If you or your staffs have any questions about this report, please contact me at (202) 512-7114 or crossem@gao.gov. Contact points for our Office of Congressional Relations and Public Affairs may be found on the last page of this report. GAO staff who made major contributions to this report are listed in appendix V.

Marcia Crosse
Director, Health Care

Appendix I: Drug Sponsors Contacted by FDA in 2008 Regarding Information on Antibiotic Labels

As one step in FDA's efforts to implement the provision in the Food and Drug Administration Amendments Act of 2007 regarding antibiotic effectiveness, FDA identified 210 antibiotics for which sponsors were responsible for evaluating and maintaining and, if necessary, updating the breakpoints on their antibiotics' labels. In January and February of 2008, FDA sent letters to the sponsors of these drugs reminding them of the importance of regularly updating the breakpoints on their antibiotic labels. In addition, the letters requested that sponsors evaluate and maintain the currency of breakpoints included on their labels and within 30 days submit evidence to FDA showing that the breakpoints were either current or needed revision. Of the 210 antibiotics, 126 were brand-name antibiotics and 84 were generic antibiotics, manufactured by 39 different sponsors. Table 2 identifies these 39 sponsors and whether the sponsor held a brand-name antibiotic, a generic antibiotic, or both.

Table 2: Drug Sponsors Receiving Letters from FDA in 2008 in Response to the Food and Drug Administration Amendments Act of 2007 Regarding Information on Antibiotic Labels

Drug sponsor	Sponsor held brand-name antibiotic	Sponsor held generic antibiotic
Abbott	X	X
APP	X	X
Astellas	X	X
AstraZeneca	X	
B. Braun	X	X
Baxter	X	X
Bayer	X	
Boehringer Ingelheim		X
Bristol-Myers Squbb	X	X
Cornerstone	X	
Cubist	X	
DAVA		X
Depomed	X	
Forest	X	
GlaxoSmithKline	X	X
Hospira	X	X
JHP	X	
Johnson & Johnson	X	
King	X	X
Lupin		X

Drug sponsor	Sponsor held brand-name antibiotic	Sponsor held generic antibiotic
Medicis		x
Merck	x	
Mutual	x	
Mylan		x
Novartis	x	x
Par		x
Patheon		x
Pfizer	x	x
Ranbaxy		x
Roche	x	x
Sanofi-aventis	x	
Shionogi	x	
Teva	x	x
Victory	x	
ViroPharma	x	
Warner Chilcott	x	
Watson	x	
West-Ward		x
X-GEN		x

Source: FDA.

	Number of antibiotics for which specified action was taken		
	New drug applications (NDA)	Abbreviated new drug applications (ANDA)	Total
Breakpoints on antibiotic labels have been updated or confirmed to be up to date			
Label supplement submitted and approved	50	0	**50**
Current label confirmed as up to date	13	1	**14**
Subtotal	**63**	**1**	**64**
No update nor confirmation of currency has been made for breakpoints on antibiotic labels			
FDA has not yet received a submission regarding the currency of breakpoints			
No response from sponsor	3	1	**4**
Sponsor responded stating that the antibiotic has been or would soon be discontinued	2	17	**19**
Sponsor responded stating that the antibiotic has been or would soon be withdrawn	14	6	**20**
Sponsor responded with general correspondence[a]	13	22	**35**
Subtotal	**32**	**46**	**78**
Sponsor submission is under review by FDA	6	6	**12**
FDA reviewed sponsor submission and requested a revision or additional information	25	31	**56**
Subtotal	**63**	**83**	**146**
Total	**126**	**84**	**210**

Source: GAO analysis of FDA data as of November 2011.

[a]The "general correspondence" category includes all communications by sponsors that did not consist of a submission regarding the currency of breakpoints included on their antibiotics' labels or a communication that the ant biotic has been or would be withdrawn or discontinued. For example, some sponsors responded with questions about what information they needed to submit.

Appendix III: Timeline of FDA Implementation of Certain Food and Drug Administration Amendments Act Provisions

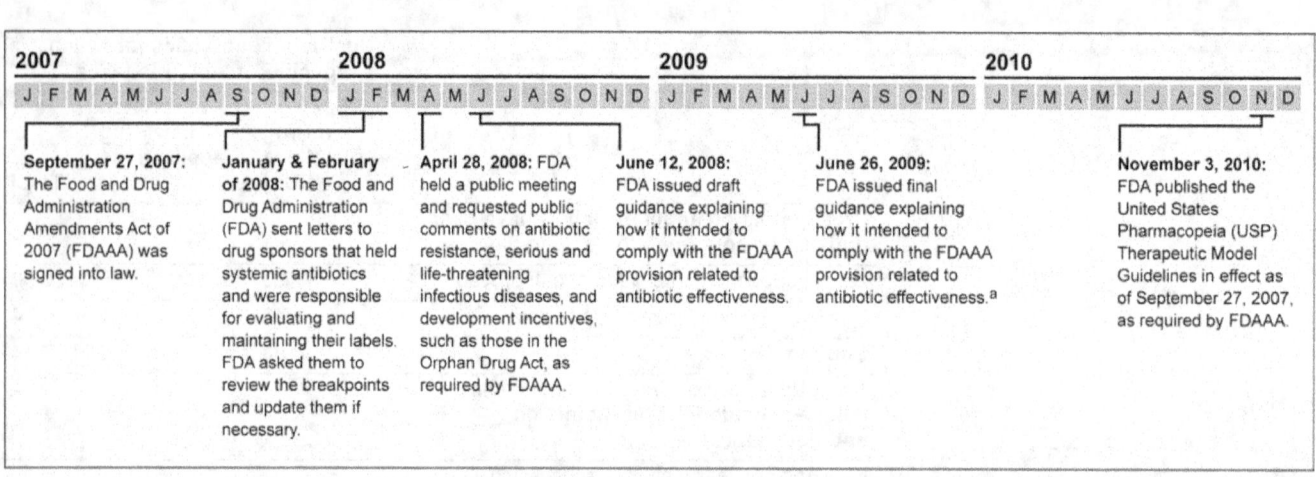

2007

J F M A M J J A S O N D

September 27, 2007: The Food and Drug Administration Amendments Act of 2007 (FDAAA) was signed into law.

2008

J F M A M J J A S O N D

January & February of 2008: The Food and Drug Administration (FDA) sent letters to drug sponsors that held systemic antibiotics and were responsible for evaluating and maintaining their labels. FDA asked them to review the breakpoints and update them if necessary.

April 28, 2008: FDA held a public meeting and requested public comments on antibiotic resistance, serious and life-threatening infectious diseases, and development incentives, such as those in the Orphan Drug Act, as required by FDAAA.

June 12, 2008: FDA issued draft guidance explaining how it intended to comply with the FDAAA provision related to antibiotic effectiveness.

2009

J F M A M J J A S O N D

June 26, 2009: FDA issued final guidance explaining how it intended to comply with the FDAAA provision related to antibiotic effectiveness.[a]

2010

J F M A M J J A S O N D

November 3, 2010: FDA published the United States Pharmacopeia (USP) Therapeutic Model Guidelines in effect as of September 27, 2007, as required by FDAAA.

Source: GAO analysis of FDA information.

[a]See FDA, *Guidance for Industry: Updating Labeling for Susceptibility Test Information in Systemic Antibacterial Drug Products and Antimicrobial Susceptibility Testing Devices* (June 2009).

Appendix IV: Comments from the Department of Health and Human Services

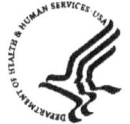 DEPARTMENT OF HEALTH & HUMAN SERVICES

OFFICE OF THE SECRETARY

Assistant Secretary for Legislation
Washington, DC 20201

Marcia Crosse
Director, Health Care
U.S. Government Accountability Office
441 G Street NW
Washington, DC 20548

DEC 1 9 2011

Dear Ms. Crosse:

Attached are comments on the U.S. Government Accountability Office's (GAO) draft report entitled, "ANTIBIOTICS: FDA Needs to Do More to Ensure that Drug Labels Contain Up-to-Date Information" (GAO 12-218).

The Department appreciates the opportunity to review this report before its publication.

Sincerely,

Jim R. Esquea
Assistant Secretary for Legislation

Attachment

**GENERAL COMMENTS OF THE DEPARTMENT OF HEALTH AND HUMAN
SERVICES (HHS) ON THE GOVERNMENT ACCOUNTABILITY OFFICE'S (GAO)
DRAFT REPORT ENTITLED, "ANTIBIOTICS: FDA NEEDS TO DO MORE TO
ENSURE THAT DRUG LABELS CONTAIN UP-TO-DATE INFORMATION" (GAO-12-
218)**

The Department appreciates the opportunity to comment on this draft report.

The Food and Drug Administration (FDA) views the updating of breakpoints for antibacterial
drugs as an important area of work and is committed to continuing its efforts to ensure that
breakpoint information is up-to-date. The agency acknowledges the importance of the issues that
GAO has identified and indeed has been working very hard to address the concerns GAO raises.
In fact, FDA already has taken steps to expedite the review of sponsor submissions regarding
breakpoints for antibacterial drugs and obtain breakpoint information from sponsors that have
not yet submitted information in response to the 2008 letters from the agency. Furthermore,
FDA also has reminded sponsors on numerous occasions of their responsibility to evaluate and
maintain up to date breakpoints. The agency will consider all of GAO's recommendations as it
continues to improve its processes to ensure that antibacterial drug labels contain up-to-date
breakpoint information.

However, FDA is concerned that GAO's report does not fully capture the breadth of both FDA's
efforts and the challenges associated with updating the labels of antibacterial drugs. We provide
the following context for this draft report.

The Food and Drug Administration Amendments Act (FDAAA) was signed into law in 2007.
Section 1111 of FDAAA requires FDA to identify and periodically update susceptibility test
interpretive criteria for antibacterial drug products and to make those findings publicly
available.[1] In order to address this provision in FDAAA, the agency took several steps as
described below.

The agency sent letters to holders of certain antibacterial drug applications reminding them of the
need to keep their drug product breakpoint information up-to-date and asking each firm for its
plan to do so. In order to establish a streamlined process for industry and the agency to conduct
this work, FDA published, a "Draft Guidance for Industry: Updating Labeling for Susceptibility
Test Information in Systemic Antibacterial Drug Products and Antimicrobial Susceptibility
Testing Devices" (breakpoints guidance) in June 2008. It described two general approaches that
companies could use to update breakpoint information in drug product labeling:

1. A more traditional approach, in which a company submits data in a labeling supplement
    that is then reviewed by the agency.[2]

2. A second approach, in which FDA would pre-review and publicly recognize (by
    publication in the Federal Register) individual drug and organism-specific susceptibility
    testing standards established by a nationally or internationally recognized standard

---

[1] FDAAA (Public Law 110-85) available at: http://www.gpo.gov/fdsys/pkg/PLAW-110publ85/pdf/PLAW-
110publ85.pdf
[2] The breakpoints guidance describes this approach in the context of when the sponsor believes that breakpoints
different from the FDA recognized standard are appropriate for their product. It is also consistent with the general
approach of submitting a labeling supplement with scientific data to support a labeling change.

1

GENERAL COMMENTS OF THE DEPARTMENT OF HEALTH AND HUMAN
SERVICES (HHS) ON THE GOVERNMENT ACCOUNTABILITY OFFICE'S (GAO)
DRAFT REPORT ENTITLED, "ANTIBIOTICS: FDA NEEDS TO DO MORE TO
ENSURE THAT DRUG LABELS CONTAIN UP-TO-DATE INFORMATION" (GAO-12-
218)

development organization. Companies would then have the option of simply submitting
labeling in compliance with the standard.

FDA expected that the traditional approach of submitting a labeling supplement with scientific
data to support a breakpoint change would be difficult for many sponsors to undertake,
particularly firms that may not have clinical microbiology expertise. The FDA standards
recognition process described in the second approach would allow companies with little
expertise and resources to use scientifically sound, already FDA accepted standards, serve
multiple firms who manufacture similar drugs with the same active ingredient (e.g., ampicillin),
and avoid having each firm individually locate scientific data on how susceptibility patterns have
evolved over time. In addition, the second approach would be a resource for firms that may not
have clinical microbiology expertise.

FDA finalized the breakpoint guidance in June 2009.[3] The agency held a public Anti-Infective
Drugs Advisory Committee Meeting on September 26, 2009 to get advice from the Committee
on implementation of the procedures described in the guidance document and to provide
information to stakeholders, including drug companies that market antibacterial drugs.

Soon after the September 2009 Advisory Committee meeting, FDA received a Congressional
letter that expressed serious concern about the propriety of FDA's use of the standards set by
nationally or internationally recognized standard development organizations as described in
FDA's breakpoints guidance. The letter also raised concerns about industry participation in the
process of an outside organization setting the breakpoints. At this time, the agency shifted focus
to work with companies to update labels for individual antibacterial drug products, using the
traditional approach (i.e., by submission of individual labeling supplements for each drug
application), as a practical way to continue making progress while the agency addressed the
concerns raised by the Congressional letter.

On February 4, 2010, FDA responded to the Congressional letter, explaining that the agency
retains ultimate authority to either accept or reject standards set by nationally or internationally
recognized standard development organizations, and that FDA will work with such organizations
to promote transparency of procedures, evaluation of potential conflicts of interest, and the
availability to the public of scientific explanations for changes to a standard. FDA asserted in its
response that the process described in its guidance document and discussed at the Advisory
Committee Meeting provides a means to appropriately update the labeling of antibacterial drugs.
FDA continues to believe that the standards recognition process is an appropriate and feasible
way to update breakpoints, and it may utilize this process in the future.

Since 2009, a number of companies have submitted labeling supplements for their drug products
(i.e., a traditional approach), and these supplements have varied in quality and completeness.

---

[3] Guidance for Industry: Updating Labeling for Susceptibility Test Information in Systemic Antibacterial Drug
Products and Antimicrobial Susceptibility Testing Devices. (June 2009). available at:
http://www.fda.gov/downloads/Drugs/GuidanceComplianceRegulatoryInformation/Guidances/UCM169359.pdf

2

**GENERAL COMMENTS OF THE DEPARTMENT OF HEALTH AND HUMAN
SERVICES (HHS) ON THE GOVERNMENT ACCOUNTABILITY OFFICE'S (GAO)
DRAFT REPORT ENTITLED, "ANTIBIOTICS: FDA NEEDS TO DO MORE TO
ENSURE THAT DRUG LABELS CONTAIN UP-TO-DATE INFORMATION" (GAO-12-
218)**

Unfortunately, many submissions contain data that have been insufficient for FDA to arrive at
updated breakpoints. FDA also notes that some companies have provided quality submissions
leading to appropriate updates of their labels.

As of December 12, 2011, the labeling for 66 antibacterial drugs has been updated or found to be
correct. The agency has developed a public website that lists the systemic antibacterial drugs
that have had their breakpoints updated, or were found to be up-to-date, and the date of the
assessment.[4] FDA expects this information will be useful to those interested in breakpoints.
FDA also has a system for tracking such work and will soon be able to do so using its internal
FDA electronic administrative record keeping system.

The GAO report also notes some areas of either incorrect or incomplete knowledge on the part of
some companies that they interviewed. It is critical that companies understand their
responsibilities for keeping their antibacterial drug product labeling up-to-date, and that they
submit labeling supplements with adequate data in order to update or keep antibacterial drug
product labeling up-to-date. FDA has provided information to stakeholders on the topic of
breakpoints and updating breakpoints through the previously mentioned breakpoints guidance
document, a draft guidance document on submitting microbiological data for systemic
antibacterial drugs,[5] the October 26, 2009 FDA Anti-Infective Drugs Advisory Committee
Meeting, interactions with sponsors in the setting of reviewing labeling supplements, and
through presentations and attendance at scientific meetings on this topic. FDA looks forward to
continued interactions with companies as they continue their efforts to update their drug product
labeling.

FDA has invested considerable time and effort over the last few years to update breakpoints.
Evaluating and updating breakpoints is challenging, however. Before one can assess a
breakpoint in product labeling, one needs to have data on the current breakpoint and how it is
performing. Unfortunately, currently relevant and adequate scientific data to assess a breakpoint
are not always available. When such data are not available from the drug sponsor, agency
reviewers search the literature and query the archives of standard development organizations to
identify such data. In some instances these efforts are successful, and in other cases the search
may not yield data to address the question at hand. Even a successfully updated breakpoint may
need to be updated as circumstances evolve. Despite these challenges, the agency is committed
to the important public health goal of updating antibacterial drug breakpoints, and looks forward
to continued progress in this area.

---

[4] FDA website on Antibacterial Product Labeling: Microbiology Susceptibility Interpretive Criteria (Breakpoints)
and Quality Control Parameter Updates. Available at:
http://www.fda.gov/AboutFDA/CentersOffices/OfficeofMedicalProductsandTobacco/CDER/ucm275763.htm
[5] Draft Guidance for Industry: Microbiological Data for Systemic Antibacterial Drug Products — Development,
Analysis, and Presentation. (September 2009). available at:
http://www.fda.gov/downloads/Drugs/GuidanceComplianceRegulatoryInformation/Guidances/UCM182288.pdf

3

Appendix V: GAO Contact and Staff Acknowledgments

GAO Contact	Marcia Crosse, (202) 512-7114 or crossem@gao.gov
Staff Acknowledgments	In addition to the contact named above, Geri Redican-Bigott, Assistant Director; Alison Binkowski; Ashley R. Dixon; Cathleen Hamann; Lisa Motley; Patricia Roy; Laurie F. Thurber; and Jocelyn Yin made key contributions to this report.

www.ingramcontent.com/pod-product-compliance
Lightning Source LLC
Chambersburg PA
CBHW080926290526
45795CB00007BA/2670